Isometric Exercise Guide

A Complete Step-By-Step Guide For Building Muscle And Strength Through Isometric Exercises

Vicky Klocko

Table of Contents

CHAPTER ONE

Introduction

Isometric exercises form a unique category in the realm of fitness. Unlike traditional exercises that involve joint movement, isometric exercises focus on muscle contractions without altering the length of the muscle or the angle of the joints. In simpler terms, you're essentially holding a position without movement, activating specific muscles to generate force against an immovable object or by tensing the muscles themselves.

The benefits of isometric exercises are diverse. They're excellent for building strength, enhancing stability, and improving muscular endurance. Due to their nature, isometric exercises can be especially useful in rehabilitation settings, helping maintain or rebuild muscle strength without excessive strain on recovering joints or tissues.

These exercises require minimal to no equipment and can be easily integrated into various routines. Popular examples include planks, wall sits, and certain yoga poses that emphasize holding positions and engaging specific muscle groups for an extended period.

Isometric exercises are versatile, accessible, and can complement dynamic workouts, contributing to a well-rounded fitness regimen. They're also adaptable to different fitness levels, making them suitable for beginners and advanced athletes alike.

Understanding Isometric Exercises

Isometric exercises involve muscle contractions without joint movement. This means the muscle generates tension and strength without actually lengthening or shortening. You're essentially holding a static position, activating specific muscles against resistance. This resistance could be your body weight, an immovable object, or even just the tension you create within the muscle itself.

Benefits of Isometric Training

Strength Building: Isometric exercises target specific muscles and can lead to significant strength gains. They challenge muscles in a unique way, promoting muscle fiber recruitment and overall strength development.

Joint Stability: These exercises enhance joint stability by engaging the surrounding muscles without subjecting the joints to excessive movement or stress.

Injury Rehabilitation: Isometrics are often used in rehabilitation programs. They allow individuals to strengthen muscles around injured areas without putting strain on the injured tissues or joints.

Time Efficiency: Isometric exercises can be efficient, as they often require minimal time and equipment. They can be done almost anywhere, making them accessible for busy schedules.

Versatility: They can be tailored to various fitness levels and easily integrated into different routines, whether as standalone exercises or as part of a broader workout program.

Blood Pressure Regulation: Some research suggests that isometric exercises may aid in regulating blood pressure, although it's important to consult a healthcare professional for guidance on this.

These benefits make isometric exercises a valuable addition to a well-rounded fitness regimen, offering targeted strength gains, joint stability, and versatility in training routines.

Upper Body Isometric Exercises
Wall Push:

Method: Stand arm's length away from a sturdy wall, place your palms against it at shoulder height. Push against the wall without moving, engaging your chest, shoulders, and triceps.

Process: Hold the position for a set duration, maintaining a steady pressure against the wall.

Plank:

Method: Get into a push-up position, but instead of supporting yourself on your hands, rest your forearms on the ground. Keep your body in a straight line, engaging your core, shoulders, and back.

Process: Hold the plank position, ensuring your body remains straight and aligned, without sagging or lifting the hips excessively, for a specific duration.

Static Arm Curls:

Method: Hold a dumbbell or any weight in each hand, with arms bent at 90 degrees.

Process: Keep the arms in that position, engaging the biceps without moving the elbows or curling the weights. Maintain the contraction for the desired duration.

Lower Body Isometric Exercises

Wall Sit:

Method: Lean against a wall and slide down until your knees are bent at a 90-

degree angle, as if you were sitting in an imaginary chair.

Process: Hold this position, engaging your quads, hamstrings, and glutes, keeping your back against the wall for the intended duration.

Static Squat:

Method: Assume a squat position with feet shoulder-width apart, knees bent at 90 degrees, and back straight.

Process: Hold the squat position without moving up or down, engaging your quadriceps, hamstrings, and glutes.

Calf Raises against a Wall:

Method: Stand facing a wall with your hands resting against it for balance, and rise onto the balls of your feet.

Process: Hold the raised position, engaging your calf muscles, without lowering your heels for the desired duration.

CHAPTER TWO
Core Isometric Exercises

Plank Variations:

Method: Vary the plank by lifting one arm or leg, adding instability by using an exercise ball, or performing side planks.

Process: Maintain the modified plank positions, engaging core muscles to stabilize the body for the specified time.

Abdominal Bracing:

Method: Lie on your back, tighten your abdominal muscles as if preparing to be punched in the stomach.

Process: Hold this tightened position, engaging the core muscles, without holding your breath.

Side Plank:

Method: Lie on your side, supporting your body with one forearm and the side of your foot.

Process: Hold the position with your body in a straight line, engaging the obliques and core muscles on the side facing the ground.

Full Body Isometric Exercises

Superman Pose:

Method: Lie face down on the floor, extend arms in front and lift both arms and legs simultaneously.

Process: Hold the lifted position, engaging the back, glutes, and shoulders, without arching excessively.

Static Lunge:

Method: Step forward into a lunge position, bending both knees at 90 degrees.

Process: Hold the lunge position, engaging quadriceps, hamstrings, and glutes without moving up or down.

Bridge Pose:

Method: Lie on your back, bend your knees, and lift your hips off the ground.

Process: Hold the raised position, engaging the glutes, hamstrings, and lower back muscles without lowering your hips.

These exercises, when performed correctly and consistently, offer a diverse range of isometric workouts targeting various muscle groups, contributing to overall strength, stability, and muscular endurance.

Shoulders and Arms Isometric Exercises

Isometric Shoulder Press:

Method: Hold a pair of dumbbells at shoulder height with elbows bent at 90 degrees.

Process: Push the weights upward against an immovable object (such as a door frame or wall) while maintaining the elbow angle.

Isometric Bicep Curl:

Method: Hold a dumbbell or resistance band in one hand, elbow bent at 90 degrees.

Process: Attempt to curl the weight upward while resisting the movement with the opposite hand. Swap hands to work both biceps evenly.

Chest Isometric Exercise

Isometric Chest Squeeze:

Method: Hold a yoga block, medicine ball, or a cushion between your palms at chest level.

Process: Squeeze the object with maximum force without allowing it to move. Maintain the pressure for the desired duration.

Back Isometric Exercise

Isometric Pull:

Method: Attach a resistance band to a stationary object at chest height.

Process: Hold the ends of the band and pull it towards your body, engaging your back muscles, while keeping the band stationary.

Full Body Isometric Exercises

Horse Stance:

Method: Stand with feet wider than shoulder-width apart, squat down until thighs are parallel to the ground.

Process: Hold the squat position, engaging thighs, glutes, and core, maintaining the posture without standing up.

Plank with Leg Lift:

Method: Start in a plank position.

Process: Lift one leg a few inches off the ground while keeping your body stable and level. Alternate legs for an isometric challenge to the core and glutes.

Isometric Deadlift Hold:

Method: Stand with a barbell or pair of dumbbells in hand.

Process: Lower the weights as if performing a deadlift, pause halfway and hold the position for a specific duration before returning to the starting position.

These exercises target specific muscle groups, offering a comprehensive range of isometric workouts for a full-body engagement, helping to build strength, stability, and muscular endurance. Incorporating these exercises into a routine can provide a well-rounded isometric training regimen.

Isometric Exercises with Equipment

Resistance Band Holds:

Method: Anchor a resistance band to a stable object at ground level or higher.

Process: Hold the band with both hands and create tension by pulling in different directions, maintaining the hold against the resistance for the desired duration. Examples include chest press holds, row holds, or overhead press holds.

Isometric Holds with Dumbbells:

Method: Hold dumbbells in various positions without movement.

Process: Perform static holds in exercises like the static lunge hold, isometric bicep curl hold, or isometric overhead press hold. Hold the weights at a specific angle, engaging muscles without performing the full range of motion.

Stability Ball Exercises:

Method: Use a stability ball to introduce instability into isometric exercises.

Process: Perform exercises such as stability ball planks, stability ball wall squats, or stability ball hamstring curls. These exercises engage core stability while working specific muscle groups.

TRX Suspension Trainer Holds:

Method: Adjust the TRX straps to perform isometric holds.

Process: Engage in exercises like TRX chest press holds or TRX squat holds, maintaining the position against the resistance provided by the suspension trainer.

Barbell Isometric Holds:

Method: Load a barbell with weight and hold specific positions without movement.

Process: Perform isometric exercises such as barbell rack holds (holding the barbell at a specific position in a squat or deadlift), engaging muscles to stabilize against the weight.

Kettlebell Isometric Holds:

Method: Hold kettlebells in various positions to challenge specific muscle groups.

Process: Perform exercises like kettlebell goblet squat holds, kettlebell farmer's carry holds, or kettlebell bottoms-up holds, engaging muscles to maintain control and stability.

Incorporating equipment into isometric exercises adds versatility and intensity to your workouts. These variations challenge muscles in different ways, promoting strength, stability, and control while targeting specific muscle groups. Always ensure proper form and technique to maximize the benefits of these exercises.

CHAPTER THREE

Advanced Isometric Exercises

Planche Progression:

Method: The planche is an advanced gymnastic move where the body is held parallel to the ground, supported only by the hands.

Process: Progression involves starting with tuck planche, where the body is tucked with knees close to the chest and gradually extending the legs to a full planche position. This requires tremendous upper body and core strength.

L-Sit:

Method: In an L-sit, the body is held upright, with legs extended and raised parallel to the ground while supporting yourself with your hands.

Process: Start with bent knees and gradually extend the legs, engaging the core and hip flexors intensely to hold the position.

Handstand Hold:

Method: A handstand involves balancing the body upside down on hands, with legs extended upwards.

Process: Begin against a wall for support, gradually progressing to freestanding handstands. Holding the handstand position demands substantial shoulder, core, and arm strength, along with balance and coordination.

Front Lever Progression:

Method: In a front lever, the body hangs horizontally from a bar, parallel to the ground, supported only by the arms.

Process: Progression involves gradually extending the body from tucked positions to full front lever, demanding immense upper body and core strength.

Human Flag Progression:

Method: The human flag involves holding the body horizontally sideways off a vertical pole, supported only by the arms.

Process: Progress from tuck positions to eventually holding the body straight with legs extended. This requires significant upper body, core, and oblique strength.

Back Lever Progression:

Method: In a back lever, the body hangs horizontally from a bar facing downwards, parallel to the ground.

Process: Progression involves starting with tucked positions and gradually extending the body to a full back lever, challenging the back, core, and arm muscles intensely.

These advanced isometric exercises demand exceptional strength, stability, and body awareness. They often require careful progression and proper form to avoid injury and build the necessary strength to execute the positions effectively.

Safety Tips for Isometric Exercises

Proper Breathing Techniques:

- Focus on maintaining steady breathing throughout each exercise. Avoid holding your breath, as it can increase blood pressure and limit oxygen flow. Breathe deeply and rhythmically, syncing your breath with the isometric holds.

Importance of Proper Form:

- Correct form is crucial to prevent injuries and maximize effectiveness. Ensure proper body alignment and posture during each exercise. Engage the targeted muscles without straining other body parts, and avoid arching or rounding the back.

Avoiding Overexertion:

- Gradually increase the duration or intensity of isometric holds to avoid overexertion. Pushing too hard too quickly can lead to muscle strains or injury. Listen to your body and gradually progress over time.

Conclusion

Isometric exercises offer strength building, joint stability, and are versatile for various fitness levels.They aid in rehabilitation by strengthening muscles without excessive joint stress.Isometrics can be time-efficient and require minimal equipment, making them accessible.

Also tips for Incorporating Isometric Exercises into a Routine includes:

- **Mix it Up:** Combine isometric exercises with dynamic movements for a comprehensive workout.

- **Progress Gradually:** Start with shorter holds or easier variations and gradually increase intensity or duration.

- **Consistency is Key:** Incorporate isometric exercises regularly into your routine for optimal benefits.

- **Seek Guidance:** Consult a fitness professional to ensure proper form and progression.

Isometric exercises can be a valuable addition to any fitness regimen, offering targeted strength gains, enhanced stability, and versatile workout options. Prioritizing safety, proper form, and gradual progression will help you reap the full benefits of these exercises while minimizing the risk of injury.

Isometric exercises offer a multitude of benefits that cater to various fitness goals and levels. These static holds and muscle contractions provide an effective means to build strength, improve stability, and enhance muscular endurance without the need for extensive equipment or space. The versatility of isometric exercises allows for integration into diverse workout routines, making them accessible to beginners and challenging enough for advanced fitness enthusiasts.

Their significance in rehabilitation cannot be overlooked, as isometrics facilitate muscle strengthening without subjecting injured joints or tissues to excessive strain. By incorporating proper breathing techniques, maintaining correct form, and avoiding overexertion, individuals can safely harness the benefits of isometric exercises while reducing the risk of injury.

Incorporating isometric exercises regularly into a fitness routine, gradually progressing in duration or intensity, and seeking guidance when needed from fitness professionals are key strategies for maximizing their advantages. Whether it's the foundational plank or the advanced planche progression, these exercises offer an array of options to enhance overall strength, stability, and muscular control.

Remember, consistency and proper technique are the cornerstones of successful isometric training, unlocking a pathway to improved fitness and overall well-being.

THE END